A QUAKER LOOKS AT YOGA

DOROTHY ACKERMAN
Pendle Hill Pamphlet 207

About the Author / Dorothy Ackerman has been a member of the Twin Cities Meeting in Minneapolis for the past fifteen years. She met her husband, Eugene, in the Conscientious Objector group at Brown University where she was an undergraduate in Fine Arts and he a graduate student in Physics. Their two sons, Frank and Manny, were also CO's, and their daughter Amy married a Swedish CO. Gene's scientific approach is a constant challenge and balance to Dorothy's delight in the magical. Now a retired parent and recently a grandparent, she is freeing herself from old roles and old dependencies, so that, in the words of her younger son, she will become an "Ackerperson."

Having been addicted to creativity for fifty years she is curious about the source of it all. As an artist she "tunes in" to inspiration, and as a Quaker she tunes in similarly to the Inner Light. To learn more control of the process she has looked into ESP, Mind Control, and mysticism in general, as well as Yoga. She was fortunate to have two Yoga teachers—Swami Radha and Swami Rama—who were knowledgeable about modern psychology and the research being done on meditation. During her year as a student at Pendle Hill Dorothy presented her ideas on the relationship between Quakerism and Yoga, which she has since expanded into this pamphlet.

Request for permission to quote or to translate should be addressed to Pendle Hill Publications, Wallingford, Pennsylvania 19086.

Copyright © July 1976 by Pendle Hill
ISBN 0-87574-207-6
Library of Congress catalog card number 76-23909

Printed in the United States of America by
Sowers Printing Company, Lebanon, Pennsylvania

July 1976: 3,000

One Sunday at the close of Meeting for Worship a young Friend asked whether we could get together during the week to meditate. Laughingly I asked, "Isn't that what we just finished doing?" Quietly he said, "I don't mean that; I mean really meditating!" I shared his discontent. The spiritual pulse of our Meeting was weak. There was a chronic dribbling in of latecomers and dribbling out of early leavers. Our Meeting was restless with many distractions including the reading of books.

Out of our shared longing to "really meditate" a small worship group was born which met irregularly over a period of two years whenever the need was felt and the time was auspicious. Then for one year it met concurrently with the scheduled Meeting for Worship. It was small and informal; we lay or sat on the floor, sat on cushions or chairs, whatever we preferred. As we experimented with different techniques of centering: singing, chanting, holding hands, or talking quietly together before entering the silence, we experienced an intensity of focus which is rare in our large Meeting for Worship.

This pamphlet is the result of my search for the missing ingredient. My concern is not new; thirty years ago Gerald Heard said that Friends, having failed to develop a psychology or a precise method for using the silence effectively, should blend Yoga with Quakerism. Since my own experience of the Light at a Yoga school, I, also, have wanted to combine Yogic wisdom with Quaker beliefs and experience. I include the Yogic preparations for personal meditation and relate them to Quaker worship. I have also included initiatory experiences as they occur within the Society of Friends and outside it. In presenting Yoga to Friends I am looking past the techniques for the experience which they facilitate. Only when that experience is sympathetic to Friendly tradition have I suggested the use of Yoga.

Standing on my head is not a necessary spiritual practice; looking at the world from a new angle is. When I did a headstand in the rain, the rain appeared to be rising instead of falling. I had a completely new look at my world. Ever since then I have followed the impulse to look at things upside down in imagination if not in posture. Not having had a Quaker grandmother to prepare me for silent Meeting by holding me quietly in her arms every day, as did one Friend I know, I follow Yoga instructions to get relaxed and centered in meditation.

Jesus instructed His followers to knock, and promised that their knock would be answered. It is necessary to reach out and knock. Getting in touch with the Still Small Voice should require at least as much effort as making a phone call. When I place a phone call I do not sit down and read a book, even if it is the Bible; I do not squirm and wonder how long I will have to sit still; nor do I rush through all my thoughts of the past week. Instead, I make myself comfortable, dial the number, and wait expectantly. When my friend picks up the phone I really listen to hear what she is saying so that I do not come away with just my own thoughts. I use Yoga to knock on the door, or to place that call to Spirit. In accepting the challenge of Yoga to participate and experience the results, I have found it a helpful way, but certainly not the only way.

Traditional Centering Devices

Religion has developed many ways of communicating with the Spiritual Source. When not understood, these ways have become meaningless rituals, vain repetitions. Early Friends rightly objected to a veneration of the forms themselves. They disassociated themselves from the ritual and relied on the individual initiatory experience. Are we today in danger of losing the experience because we do not reach out and knock on the door or make that call or wait expectantly?

This group "waiting on the Lord," expecting more to manifest than the assembled persons, is based in Christianity on the promise that "when two or three are gathered together, there am I in their midst." Early Quakers were clear that these souls seeking together in spiritual communion were *the* church with Christ in its midst. When they felt this had occurred they called it a "gathered Meeting;" when they felt it had not occurred they would say that the Meeting had not been "gathered." Accordingly they referred to some places of worship as "steeple houses" and their own as meeting houses. Yoga does not include this group mystique. In a group of Yogis meditating together each is alone in meditation. The concept of "Church" is western and the concept of a "gathered meeting" without a member of the clergy in charge is unique to Quakers. In traditional church services blending of the worshippers into a spiritual unity ("gathering") is facilitated by a pattern of centering devices which we call liturgy. Hymn singing, vocal prayer, responsive reading, and group recitation center the congregation vocally, while architecture, candles, altar and priest center the group visually. The more the worshippers participate in the ritual, the deeper the centering. If the whole body were involved as in dance the centering should be more intense.

The spiritual intensity experienced during group worship comes partly from the artistry of the service and partly from the group's reaching a strength beyond its own. Some people find deep joy and renewal within the liturgical framework. Though I am devoted to silent worship after the manner of

Friends occasionally I nourish the artist in me by experiencing a high church service where all the arts join together in celebration. My favorite is the Easter service at the Cathedral of St. John the Divine in New York. There I see wall-to-wall people a quarter of a mile long; I see the processional of choirs and clerics of all ages and colors; I see embroidery, gold, precious stones; I smell incense; I hear music. We all turn from the altar and face the entrance doors at the front of the church. As the huge twenty foot doors are slowly opened to greet the Risen Christ, the trumpets blast and a shiver goes through the crowd as everyone sings "Christ the Lord is Risen Today." Here I am part of living pageantry. I absorb the color, the sight, the scent and the sound; they all work together within me. Here I am not in a museum looking at one chalice, one cross, one vestment, one altar fragment, trying to imagine the rest, I am experiencing all the arts and artifacts together, purposely creating a great religious festival. I feel an excitement that overflows in joy.

Traditionally, Quakers have said, "This is a vain show." Worship becomes a show when it has spectators rather than participants. Without liturgy to help us center it takes all of our effort to reach spiritual depths rather than emptiness. Let us not be deceived; silence is no more a guarantee of spiritual experience than liturgy.

The early Friends who rejected liturgy and the clergy had a very different life style from our own. They lived in a Puritan age and shared many Puritan ideas and customs. Families prayed together, read the Bible often and went to it for guidance. Many kept spiritual diaries called journals. In addition to weekly meetings for worship, they met whenever they felt the need, and whenever a visiting Friend came to town. Children were an integral part of the Meeting since they believed that the Holy Spirit could reach children as well as adults. They did not need a priest because they were so aware of Jesus Christ sitting at the head of the Meeting. They were aware of His immediate presence in daily life also.

Their spiritual bond was a personal experience of the Light. This inner initiation did not make life easy, as it showed up all thoughts and actions which separated them from God. The ensuing struggle for perfection was called the "Lamb's War," which they all shared in one way or another. Only afterwards did they experience the Light as nurturing.

If, in comparison, our manner of learning to use the silence effectively seems contrived, it is because we live in a different era. Lacking their intimate Christianity, we can use Yoga to help us contact the Spirit by whatever name we call it. We, too, can wait expectantly.

Yoga Philosophy

The aim of both Yogic and Quaker meditation is a mystical union which involves such a strong awareness of the Source of Life that actions flow directly from the spiritual Center, and life becomes harmonious. The Sanskrit terms and Hindu imagery of Yoga can obscure from us the fact that it is a program of study and practice designed to bring about this contact with deity. A spiritual guru (teacher) guides students to their own Inner Guru (Inner Light) and accepts it as the highest authority for each person.

Yoga says that contact with the inner divinity is blocked by our subconscious which casts its shadow in front of the Light. To remove these subconscious blocks we must first become aware of them. At this point Yoga shares with Jungian psychology an interest in dreams, symbology, slips of the tongue, jokes, and body language. Yoga provides a guru and the Jungians provide a therapist to help a person deal with this material when it seems overwhelming. Both Yoga and Jungian psychology speak of the masculine and feminine within each of us and the need to find a balance between them. Yoga holds that spirit is not reached by an absence of sexuality but by a blending.

Yoga is divided into eight "limbs." These are not the limbs of a tree which we climb, but they symbolize eight skills for overcoming obstacles, just as the many limbs of Hindu deities symbolize their many aspects. These eight limbs are: abstinence, observance, posture, breath control, withdrawal of the senses, concentration, meditation, and contemplation.

Abstinence and observance are the ethical limbs of Yoga. The abstinences are non-injury, non-lying, non-theft, non-sensuality and non-greed. "Non" is used to indicate the "absence of." Thus non-injury means not hurting self or others even unintentionally. All Yoga is based on non-injury which was strongly manifested in the life of Mahatma Gandhi. Non-injury requires that personal relationships must be harmonious before meditation is possible. In Biblical terms, "settle with your brother before petitioning the Lord."

The observances of Yoga are: cleanliness, contentment, body conditioning, self-study, and attentiveness to God. Cleanliness includes both physical cleansing and its ritual significance. Contentment means recognizing the situation for what it is and working it out, not servility or apathy. Body conditioning is familiar to the West in the Hatha Yoga exercises, sometimes thought to be all of Yoga. It is neither competitive nor gymnastic; the Hatha postures are for gaining control of the physical body and for stretching the muscles prior to relaxation; they involve no strain or competition. "Ha" is Sanskrit for sun and "Tha" for moon. So "Hatha" balances the polarities; positive and negative; hot and cold; masculine and feminine; sun and moon. Yoga teaches that by breath control we can contact the Source from which we came, since breath is the link between body and soul connecting the body with its energy (Life Force). Breath control is also taught as a way of controlling body temperature and emotions; it is a physical and emotional thermostat.

Withdrawal of the senses is a tuning out of everything that distracts us from meditation. It is an everyday occurrence which we experience whenever we focus on one thing rather than another. The same attentiveness is used in meditation as in reading a book. If I sit in Meeting reading a book I deliberately close myself off from any words, thoughts, or moving of spirit which may occur. If I sit in Meeting expectantly listening I deliberately close myself to the distractions of restless bodies, busy thought, and people reading books. Ernest Wood in his book, *Practical Yoga,* defines Yogic concentration as the skill of focusing, meditation as the act of focusing, and contemplation as the step beyond meditation where beauty, truth, light or love are actually experienced, not just thought about: Being rather than Seeing.

> It is raining and as I walk
> I become thoroughly soaked
> Which is water? Which is me?
> I've lost me. Have I found God?
>
> I'm sculpting. The alabaster peels away;
> It takes shape.
> I don't see the shape; I am the shape.
> I've lost me. Have I found God?
>
> I'm listening inside,
> The Aum is very loud, it surges
> until I feel it. I am the sound.
> I've lost me. Have I found God?
>
> I enter the silence
> I become silent. I am the silence,
> I've lost me—
> but if I ask
> I break the silence, so I'll never know
> But it is the closest I've come.

Adapting Spiritual Practice

To Friends some Yoga techniques will appear novel, even bizarre, while others will appear familiar. I have chosen to describe practices which may seem difficult because they are unfamiliar, but not those which could be personally harmful in the absence of a trained teacher. In learning to know myself I have discovered my abilities and limitations, sometimes painfully. For instance, during Minnesota winters I find Hatha Yoga is feasible in the afternoon or evening but not by the dawn's early light. The pre-dawn routine was established in tropical countries where daylight hours were too hot for exercise and by celibates who did not arouse a sleeping spouse by rising early. I have found that the Lotus posture, the trademark of Yoga, is not for me. I sit cross-legged on a pillow instead. While Yoga urges a vegetarian diet, I have not deliberately eliminated meat from my diet; on occasion I eat it, but no longer enjoy it as I used to. Though I have studied with several Yoga teachers I have avoided formal discipleship under a guru, feeling that it was incompatible with my roles of wife and Quaker.

I like the sacramental approach of Yoga to body care and washing, based on the belief that the divinity within makes the body a living temple, and thus body care becomes temple maintenance. The Yoga injunction to wait an hour after eating before meditating has been helpful, for the body can be so involved with food processing that the mind has little energy left for meditation. The Yogic morning and evening review is a familiar activity often mistaken for meditation. Yoga considers reviewing the day that has passed or planning the day to come a necessary part of mental housekeeping. It can prepare for meditation but it is not meditation any more than housecleaning is sitting down and enjoying a clean house.

Practical Application

Yoga suggests having a specific time and place for daily meditation where one can be quiet and relax. It is important to be relaxed for meditation. The first swami I listened to said that relaxation was the step most often ignored by Westerners trying to meditate and it was the most important preparation. Five years and three swamis later I agreed with him. I have seen so many Yoga students who get fascinated with the exercises and neglect the relaxation. I tend to, myself. Relaxation sounds so simple, but the popularity of methods to release tension indicate otherwise: massage, hypnosis, Yoga, meditation, therapy, mind control and bio-feedback training. The practice of driving instead of walking denies our bodies their natural exercise. When I lead an active life I can relax easily just by sitting down, but if I have been sitting most of the day I will need exercise before I can relax for meditation. Otherwise my body will rebel and get what exercise it can by squirming.

Yoga traditionally uses the Hatha Yoga to prepare the body for meditation. It is helpful but not necessary; a leisurely walk will serve as well if I consciously stretch my back tall and let my arms and legs swing freely. This is a good time to review the day and quietly resolve or set aside issues that are pending. If I try to sweep anything under the rug by not dealing with it, it usually nags me for attention as soon as I start to meditate. I have an exercise for reminding myself to let go of problems during meditation. As I walk I look at an unfamiliar object, noticing how it seems to change yet remain the same as I approach it. Then I go some distance before turning around. Then I approach it again, noticing how different it seems; I need to let it go for a while to get a fresh point of view.

I can stretch indoors too: reaching out slowly to the walls, the ceiling, and the floor in that order. I think of this as reaching out to others with love, to God for inspiration, to the earth in blessing. Then I vigorously shake myself free of impediments. I always include the Hatha neck rolling which loosens the neck and shoulders where so much tension is stored. It is merely a dropping of the head forward like a rag doll and rolling it all the way around slowly three times in one direction and then three times in the other direction.

If I sit on a chair to meditate I pick one that allows my back to be straight and my knees slightly higher than the seat so it does not press into the upper leg. If it is big and deep I sit cross-legged in it or on the floor. On the floor I sit on a small cushion or rolled blanket which allows my legs to fold comfortably in front of me.

When I am comfortably settled I focus attention on my breathing. I can feel my breath, warm as I exhale and cool as I inhale, setting the rhythm of my life. My breath is such a constant companion that I take it for granted. How remarkable that it continues all day and all night! If it is irregular just my notice will cause it to become regular. Because slow breathing cools my body and calms my emotions I deliberately slow down the rhythm for meditation. Sometimes during a very peaceful meditation my breathing slows down almost to a standstill and then later returns to normal. I have noticed that this happens naturally and I do not try to manipulate it. Yoga teaches me to close my mouth and breathe through my nose so that the air that reaches my lungs will be filtered and warm.

Sometimes my hands relax easily in my lap. Sometimes I clasp them loosely. For centering I often join the tips of my thumb and first finger Yoga style. In Meeting for Worship when I consciously reach out to others and take part in the gathering of the meeting I hold my palms open and up.

Centering in Meditation

Finally I am ready to relax my mind. Too often my mind is like a TV set which has been left on so long that no one notices it. However, in order to meditate it must be quieted. So I deliberately close my eyes and focus attention on my breathing. If this is not enough I turn my closed eyes up so that they are pointed at the spot between my eyebrows while my mind is attending to my breathing. This feat usually eliminates all other thought. Thinking takes me away from the here and now: in memory to the past and in imagination to the future. I expand my awareness by setting aside the past and the future, and becoming open to new dimensions of the present.

The Seneca Indians use feelings to reach a depth beyond thought. They say that silence is a door we go through. In order to pass through silence in this way they say, "Taste, smell, and hear the silence." The Yaqui Indians of our southwest say that you must "stop the world" to meet the totality of yourself.

Ernest Wood in describing Yogic contemplation directs us to view the focal point from all sides using the five senses and then to view it from its own center. Howard Brinton brought back from Japan the image of the mind as a pool to be quieted.

Thirty-five years ago in *Pain, Sex and Time* Gerald Heard, feeling that expansion of consciousness was the next step in evolution, said that meditation was the most important practice that we could use for the development of the species. In a later book, *Training for the Life of the Spirit,* he defines meditation as "looking in the direction of Reality," gazing "at what seems to be nothing, until through the invisible radiation which we are confronting our spiritual eyes are grown." In *Phenomenon of Man* Teilhard de Chardin expresses concern that we must develop spiritually or face the fate of phylum extinction. And Gopi Krishna, a contemporary Yogic author, in his book, *Biological Basis of Religion and Genius,* suggests that meditation can actually change our bodies. He explains that nervous energy which the Yogis call Life Force actually nourishes the body cells. In a person of genius or great spirituality the cells become irradiated with this energy. Meditation is a method of increasing the flow of the Life Force within us, so that the genius or illuminated person maintains a constant supercharge of energy at a level where it is recognized by others as charisma, or seen by artists as halos.

Electroencephalographic (EEG) research suggests that in meditation we mentally shift gears to slower brain waves than usual. This slower tempo is also present in the hypnogogic state between waking and sleeping and during the creative thought of the artist. In this state there is a freedom from the past, an openness to new ideas. Inspiration cannot be familiar; it is by definition new. Meditation approached with openness stimulates creativity and becomes a way of life. When meditation is programmed it excludes growth and becomes an escape from life.

Special Techniques for Concentration

Yogis express the difficulty of harnessing mind by referring to it as a "runaway drunken monkey." This is reflected in the variety of methods offered for gaining control of mind. Of these, chanting a mantra and gazing at a candle have received more publicity than understanding. In themselves, staring at a candle or singing a phrase over and over are not unusual experiences but when suggested as techniques for quieting the mind they somehow become mysterious.

Candle Gazing: For awhile I found candle gazing very helpful for quieting, centering and visualizing the Light. I was always clear that the candle flame reflected the Divine Light and was a symbol for my subsconscious mind. With my eyes on the flame I let all other thoughts fall away and became as strongly aware of the light as I could. Closing my eyes the flame was still visible, sometimes as a light and sometimes as a brilliant doorway for me to pass through. I imagined that the flame was in me and filled me or that I became the flame.

If you ask, "Isn't candle gazing autohypnotism? Aren't you afraid that something MIGHT HAPPEN?" I answer, "Of course it is autohypnotism, and I fervently hope something will happen." I might become autohypnotized with the idea that I have a body of Light which reflects the Divine Light. Hypnotism is no stranger to the American way of life. It is a wonder to me that the same people who fear candle gazing have no hesitation about staring at a television screen. TV is a household hypnotist; advertisers are well aware that the bright screen in a darkened room provides perfect conditions for hypnotism. It is not a case of whether we are hypnotized, but by what and for what purpose. It is better to establish a strong hypnotic relationship to the Divine Light than to TV heroes, or ads.

Mantra Chanting: A mantra is a syllable, word or phrase which is used repetitively to quiet the mind. It can be chanted verbally or silently or even written. Some teachers prefer a nonsense syllable which will not start new thoughts; others use meaningful words to guide the mind. In either case, mantra is used to flood the mind, leaving room for nothing else. One can begin to appreciate the value of mantra after daily practice for a minimum of one month. Set aside a certain time every day and repeat the mantra. Start out with five minutes and increase it gradually up to fifteen minutes. A mantra is a centering device. It should be used calmly. When it has stilled the mind and fades away into a meditative silence let it go unless thoughts distract. Then use it again. But it is important to remember that mantra can be overused and blot out inspiration. God may not be able to get a word in edgewise.

Experiment with a syllable or words that you like. "Walking in the Light" is a good mantra for Quakers. I started out with "Om" enjoying the way it vibrated in different parts of my body. If you prefer "One" it is a western equivalent. Actually oming is common in the West; we call it humming. So hum if you like.

Physical Activity: Physical Activity has been used for centering since the beginning of time. Yoga uses the postures, Zen, the walking meditation, Sufis and Shakers, dancing. Early Friends walked. During their long walks from city to city they often had spiritual openings. Walking is still a good centering device. If I have a problem it helps to take it for a walk. Walking to Meeting quietly may still be the best preparation for Worship. Circle dances appear in all primitive cultures as religious ritual. Perhaps we should take more notice of the folk dancing at conferences and weekend gatherings. If any Friends have experimented with going into worship directly from the dancing, I would like to hear from them whether the feeling of celebration carried over.

If we object to ritualistic centering devices, if we protest the rigidity of using one form till it loses meaning, then we had better look to ways of loosening up the ritual of silence which we have espoused. We must not let ourselves be imprisoned even by silence, but remain open to the spontaneous moving of Spirit blowing as it will.

Meeting for Worship Requires Preparation

All these techniques have their place in preparing for group worship. Early Friends took daily spiritual practice for granted. Their journals record private prayer, Bible reading, and personal meditation. Our Book of Discipline is called the *Faith and Practice* of Friends. If the daily practice is neglected there will be much to distract the mind in Meeting for Worship.

Without a daily review or journal, happenings of the past week can turn the Meeting hour into a period of mental housecleaning. To expect more is to expect the impossible. It is difficult to listen attentively when unfinished business shouts so loudly. A room full of Friends churning through their week's activities is different from a Meeting where Friends wait expectantly for the Holy Spirit. The former can turn into a "show and tell" time or a "popcorn" meeting. This kind of sharing is necessary, but is handled more effectively in a worship-sharing format. The quality of silence which disarmed the marauding Indians in the Quaker tale, "Fierce Feathers," is not achieved in one hour a week; it takes daily preparation. The potential of Friends' Meeting is so great that it is worth taking time to do our homework: reading, problem solving, daily meditation, and prompt arrival.

For those who feel the need, Hatha Yoga and breathing exercises can be done at home before Meeting. They are not suitable in Meeting unless a small group who all do yoga together move into worship without a break. A quiet walk to Meeting will calm the mind, relax the body, and get the breathing regular. One urban Friend deliberately parks his car six blocks from the Meeting House so as not to miss the walk before Meeting. It is impossible to center down and become part of worship, all out of breath and full of anxiety. It is so simple to wait a minute or two outside of the Meeting House, and with a long slow exhalation let go of the pressures and then with a long slow inhalation fill with peace and feel the back stretch till the top of your head rubs the sky. If your neck is still tense do slow neck rolls in each direction. Then, without visiting socially, enter the Meeting room quietly and relax into the silence. Breath watching can be used effectively for centering and for gathering the group especially if Friends feel that each is a cell in the larger body of the Meeting which through each member is breathing in and sending out Spirit.

Seating Arrangements for Meeting for Worship

It is difficult to relax and sit up straight in some of our Meeting Houses. The ancient wood benches can be comfortable if the Friend is the right height and adequately padded. The old benches were functionally designed. By adding cushions without sawing off the bench legs a corresponding amount the seat height is raised. Long-legged Friends will not notice the difference. But short-legged Friends will be left with feet swinging, or propped on the bench in front, or barely touching the floor and an uncomfortable pressure behind the knees of the upper leg from the front edge of the seat.

Metal folding chairs can be rigid, and cold as well, and often get placed so close together that the Meeting is crushed rather than gathered. I take a blanket for covering metal chairs, and I make an effort to get there early enough to separate the chairs if they are too close together.

A straight back is best for meditation. Howard Brinton told us to think of our vertebrae as slats of a Venetian blind, and to mentally run a finger up and down to align them for meditation. Yoga insists on a straight back and braces it with the interlocked legs of the Lotus position. At Pendle Hill when Lanzo del Vasta, the French Catholic disciple of Gandhi, was asked his directions for meditation, he said he did not see how Friends could meditate all hunched over and with food in their stomach. Crossing his legs in front of him on the sofa, and stretching his head tall, he pointed to his back and said, "You must have a straight line between heaven and earth." Some of our benches are too narrow for sitting cross-legged; floor cushions can be made available. Will Friends accept this as a reasonable personal preference rather than a peculiarity or affectation?

Centering in Meeting

In Meeting for Worship a mantra can be used very briefly at the beginning, or better yet, on the way to Meeting. Beyond that, continued use isolates the individual Friend from the mind of the Meeting or the meeting of minds which can occur. Friends' worship is unique in being a group meditation. We have here a tremendous potential. Other meditation groups emphasize individual meditation, or follow the words of a leader; when they meet together it is parallel meditation rather than a group dynamic. Today everyone is talking about group dynamics and trying hard to understand them. In our silent Meeting for Worship we can experience the essence of this dynamic without any camouflage.

Latecomers are the greatest obstacle to gathering or centering. I include in this the practice of having latecomers pour in when the children leave. If there are two rooms available, why not close one door at a certain time and let that group go forward in their worship uninterrupted? Why not let those who come later settle in the second room and continue their worship without getting up and moving into another room? Thus there would be two worship groups, one starting before the other with the advantages of less interruption and smaller size.

Meditation in Meeting for Worship can begin with a seed thought, or without, or it can be an attitude of listening. If you bring the seed thought, don't bring it in a book. Bring it mentally so that spirit can work on it. If a quotation is so important that it belongs in Meeting then share it with the whole group, otherwise it is divisive, cutting the reader off from the gathered Meeting. A long written selection is often too complicated for a seed; one word, one thought, one Bible verse, one line of poetry is enough. The tree will grow; we do not need to begin with it.

Some Friends have the habit of silently blessing each member or holding them in the Light. But then at some point it is important to let go and assume a listening attitude and become receptive to the spirit in the group.

Intensity of spirit does not necessarily flow from a small group. Some large Meetings become closely gathered, while some small ones fall apart. Nor does intensity require hard times; while it flourishes under persecution, it is not absent when life is comfortable.

Speaking in Meeting

Preparation for Worship does not mean coming to Meeting with a prepared message or program for personal meditation. It means coming ready to be open because God speaks directly to and through each of us. It is as though each of us is a single facet on a giant telescope mirror; each reflects part of the whole; the perfect attunement of each is necessary to the vision of the whole image. A gathered Meeting is relaxed and attentive, calm and expectant. Perhaps the tension between these opposites makes the Light glow.

Early Friends did not believe in the power of silence so much as they realized the inadequacy of the spoken word to convey spiritual truth. The power of the Lord which they called "Light" could be felt in the silence, and sometimes overflowed into words, but it was not dependent on words. It had strength to lead the Meeting without words. In the 17th century Friends were not so dependent on books as we are and were used to turning to the Lord directly for guidance. When moved, they could speak from the heart, not just the head, understanding that God needed their minds, their knowledge, everything they had within them to speak the Word. Too many times we sit waiting for something from the invisible God out there which cannot manifest unless we use the God within us to let it out. Without God we miss our potential; without us God is not manifest.

Vocal ministry at its best can be the seed of Spirit which grows and flows through the Meeting; at its worst it can be an intrusion into an otherwise nurturing silence. I like to treat another's vocal ministry as I would a thought of my own, accepting it in a relaxed fashion. If it is valid for me it will grow. I do not need to reject it or grab it in my teeth and run away with it. Perhaps the statement was sufficient; perhaps it speaks to another; perhaps it is a mistake. I can learn from mistakes, too.

A brief message leaves more room for growth than a sermon. We seek a seed, not a full grown tree. One of the most meaningful Meetings for Worship I have attended was a meeting where the first speaker spoke sincerely and falteringly, and sat down at a loss for words with which to finish. That seed grew and flowered greatly. Short parables are rich because they challenge the listener to apply them to life.

Stan Zielinski in his Pendle Hill pamphlet, *Psychology and Silence,* says that Meeting for Worship is composed of silence, communion, and the message. Silence alone, or silence and communion, can make a good Meeting, "However, when the message precedes the other stages of the Meeting we have the wagon before the horse. Then we have at best a discussion on an intellectual level, and at worst a free-for-all competition in making speeches." He mentions the spiritual bond among members and the sequence of messages, "It is as if one person were trying in a leisurely manner to solve a problem not so much by thinking as by intuition." I am reminded of Howard Thurman's first experience in Quaker Meeting. He felt strongly inspired to speak but desisted because he was a visitor and a Protestant minister and thought it unfitting. As he held back he was startled to hear a Friend get up and say his first sentence and then sit down. After awhile another Friend stood and gave his second sentence and sat down. And so it continued until his whole message had been given. I was impressed by the wonder in Howard Thurman's voice while he relived the experience.

Gathering brings us into spiritual communion, the state of being together rather than seeing each other. A Gathered Meeting is like an orchestra playing a symphony of silence without a score. Improvisation requires each player to be alert to the flow of harmony in the group. No one can play for self alone; each note must relate to the whole. Sometimes a theme is verbalized. Later it may return in variation. There may be a second theme and a third combining the first two. This group creation flows from the personality of that Meeting. It cannot be contrived or programmed.

Initiation

Quakers have shied away from formal initiations, but early Friends did not lack initiatory experiences. These came in the form of upsurges of power, expanded awareness, and personal revelation. George Fox's journal tells more than once of the Lord, or a voice, or Jesus Christ speaking to him. He also speaks of receiving strength and healing power.

Our Society of Friends was built on great expectations of the nearness of God and Christ to each individual and the resulting potential. Today in our pursuit of knowledge we hesitate to expect anything unusual. If anything extraordinary occurs we hurry to categorize it, and if we cannot, then we doubt our senses. Today when a person hears voices the tendency is to diagnose rather than listen. Thus we cut ourselves off from revelations. Can we again get in touch with this feeling of expectancy? Dare we move into a new space? Initiation means experiencing something new! This takes courage, faith, and support. Our Society of Friends can be a supportive fellowship for those going through the initiations of life.

Formal initiations recognized by our Society are membership, marriage, and memorials. A Quaker memorial service expands my awareness of the deceased as I take part in the sharing of memories. Marriage "after the manner of Friends" has been creatively adapted in recent years to be a meaningful celebration of a life initiation. The deliberations of the Committee on Clearness for marriage often brings insight to the marriage relationships of the committee members as well as of the couple which is seeking the meeting's approval. It is real challenge to sit on such a committee today.

Accepting New Members

The procedure of accepting new members into Meeting is not always straightforward. There is a tendency to say "yes" to anyone who asks, and to feel embarrassed at any hesitation. During thirty years in the Society of Friends I have heard of only two applicants being refused membership, but I have often heard of meetings being burdened with members who monopolize the worship hour or manipulate the business meeting. Friends revel in speaking truth to power in high places but hesitate to speak to aggression in their midst. The initial interview with applicants is the time to explain about the spontaneity of the unprogammmed Meeting for Worship, about God speaking through others as well as oneself, and how in Business Meeting it is within Quaker tradition to agree to disagree yet not to obstruct group action. This is more appropriate as initiatory instruction than as criticism or resentment later on. If necessary, a new member can be gently reminded of these initial remarks by an older Friend. It should be made clear that the Meeting for Worship is the well from which our social witness springs. Our history is not of a Society divided into mystics and activists but of a people whose mystical fervor drove them into fearless actions. Meetings wishing to clarify these issues with all or part of their membership would do well to look at the material prepared for this purpose by Rachel DuBois.

Coming of Age

Emotional preparation for adult responsibility and the physical changes of puberty were an important part of initiatory tradition. This continues, symbolically at least, in Christian confirmation and in Jewish Bar Mitzvah. The original inhabitants of our continent, the Amerinds, also offered tribal instruction to their adolescents. Though the customs varied from tribe to tribe they all involved the initiate's withdrawal into solitude. Quakers have no such formal tradition. It may well be that we should give more consideration to the special needs of adolescent Friends. Many of the challenges which come at puberty continue through life. We can err in making the Friendly way appear too easy and to lose our young to the demands of a stricter discipline. Our own tradition has much to offer but it fails to challenge when we do not witness to our beliefs. It is easy for young Friends to assume that older Friends either feel perfected or have given up the struggle; in either case there is not much of an invitation. A sharing of the problems, successes, and failures which beset us as adults can be a sharing of our humanity and a friendly gesture towards young Friends. One occasion for doing this might be an exchange, a sharing of journal entries; another might be spending a day of silence and fasting together ending with a sharing out of the silence.

For several years Earlham College has had a "solo" experience available as a retreat for incoming students, one of several electives offered during the late summer before fall classes begin. This program offers an experience in solitude which group members experience simultaneously. Could this be called a "gathered" solitude? Several days are spent outdoors in a wilderness area where participants are given room enough to each be alone. This provides an opportunity to reach a deep quiet and a close contact with nature. It makes a deep impression on the participants, who seem to gain both personal strength and attachment to the group. This is carefully prepared for by Outward Bound, an organization which gives specialized training in wilderness survival. It may appear a bit contrived, but it is not easy today to find that kind of solitude, nor even the solitude experienced by early Friends while walking from city to city.

Friends might like to consider a variation of this solo to fit their own needs and abilities. It would take a lot of careful preparation but it sounds well worth it. I am not suggesting this as a required initiation, nor a programmed vision but as an option. Individualistic as Friends are, I would expect that the personal experiences would range from ecological to mystical since solitude and nature speak to each person differently. If there are Friends who have experimented in this area I would be interested in sharing their evaluation of the experience.

Support Groups as a Meeting Resource

We have within our Meeting a different resource for inner strength. This is the small support group of eight to ten people who meet regularly over an extended period for the intimate sharing which is not possible in a committee of the whole, which includes our worship, business, and committee meetings and potluck suppers. In an intimate group we can find sympathy for celebration of the daily initiations which force us to change and grow. Without a pastor or a guru, Friends can minister to each other as we go through our modern version of the Lamb's War.

As spiritual awareness expands, it is beneficially shared with an intimate group of Friends. While sharing, it becomes obvious that each one has a personal glimpse of the truth rather than any one having *the* truth. Each Friend's view extends the group vision. Our belief that the Inner Light can shine through each of us is a reminder that the power we begin to realize as we grow spiritually is not ours to be used selfishly; rather, it is divine, as we act as stewards or channels.

A support group whose members choose to be honest is helpful in warding off the false humility which takes pride in self-denigration. If we really believe in the Inner Light, and accept George Fox's statement that we are living temples of Spirit, then it is dishonest to deny our potential. There is no need for embarrassment in sharing inspired thoughts, nor honest self-evaluation. Personal revelations require an honest and loving response from group members; silence, hostility, or cynicism are not adequate responses. Real sharing, listening, and responding are called for.

A natural sharing of hopes and fears, successes and failures, evaluation and reassurance goes on between close friends. However, sometimes one person's needs are too great for another to share alone. Also new attenders at Meeting may have a special need for support until they get well acquainted. Defeats do come in life, and then support is needed most. When a much loved Friend took his own life we, the survivors, wondered what we could or should have done. A small ongoing support group can help in times of crisis because it has shared the hopes and fears. Too often our concern comes too late. Not only would this be an extended family relationship but it could also act as a personal Clearness Committee when individuals need help in decision making.

Spiritual and Artistic Resources

Concern for the initiatory process, like interest in the techniques of Yoga, is a move towards resanctifying life as our world becomes depleted. As Friends, when we discarded the liturgy we lost Gregorian chants; when we spurned "steeplehouses" we lost stained glass windows; when we rejected the church calendar we lost the Christian metaphor of the changing seasons. Simplicity need not be sterile or ugly. With our expanded view of world history and religion there is a wealth of spiritual nourishment available. Our lives can become rich; we can select from the East and the West, from Yoga and the Amerinds. Worship can overflow into rejoicing and celebration, even into dance! Why not?

The artist in me is too strong to turn my back on beauty. I am a spiritual pack rat with an attic full of treasures from all over the world. I want my spiritual life meaningful so I will carefully select those things which complement and interpret each other. Your choices will not be the same as mine. Within me is a Presbyterian, a Congregationalist, an Episcopalian, a would-be Franciscan, a Quaker, a Yogi, an artist and a therapist in training and more. I stand at the crossroads of culture; it feels like Grand Central Station, a confusing place to be if I do not know where I am going. If, however, I know my destination, it is a convenient spot from which to make connections.

From Yoga I have learned how to sit, to breathe and relax in meditation. From the Buddhists I learned to watch my breath. From my Presbyterian childhood I became familiar with the Bible and with Jesus as a friend. From the Episcopalians I learned that truth can be robed in splendor. From Quakers I learned that truth can be simple and known directly today by each one of us. From the Amerinds I learned a reverence for the sacredness of this land, where I, too, may expect visions.

From the Congregationalists I learned the autonomy of each congregation being a community in itself. From the Franciscans I learned that life can be dedicated and severe, but beautiful. The therapist in training says, "Be open to new experiences. Don't limit yourself by cultural or family types. Know yourself; recognize the blocks to meditation, whether they be anger, pride, or fear. Know them so you can deal with them." The artist weaves all this together. As I walk the path of initiation with other seekers I bring my riches to share, and they bring theirs, and we are all enriched. In Meeting for Worship I use all I have to tune in to the Presence which I call the Christ Consciousness or the Inner Light. The challenge requires me to make wise and discriminating use of all my skills and all my treasures.

Questions for Quakers

1. In planning our Meeting rooms do we consider what physical arrangements help, rather than hinder, relaxed meditation? Do we provide low chairs or foot rests for short-legged Friends? Do we provide space for those who prefer to sit cross-legged? Do we provide breathing space between bodies? What do we do about latecomers?
2. Do we provide instruction for new members and attenders who are beginners in silent meditation? What provision do we make for helping them handle the blocks to meditation as these surface from the subconscious?
3. Are we doing our daily homework? Can we earn the Yogic beatitude, "Blessed is the human life in which there has been so much real thinking or meditation that there remains nothing scattered about, but the whole mind is redolent of unity?
4. Do we have enough confidence in the Inner Light to take what is helpful from other traditions without fear of endangering Quakerism?
5. Do we believe that a gathered Meeting depends on chance? on preparation? on grace? on the size of the group? on the familiarity of members? What, if anything, can we do to facilitate gathering?
6. Do we apply the Quaker practice of centering down and gathering in our personal life from day to day? in our meetings? in our committees? in our conferences?
7. Do we accept joy and humor as spiritual gifts? Are we open to joyous expression of praise and celebration in Meeting for Worship? What if this takes the form of laughter, song, or dance?

Bibliography

ABOUT YOGA

Krishna, Gopi. *Biological Basis of Religion and Genius.* Harper and Row, New York, 1971. An interesting explanation of genius, charisma, and spirituality by a contemporary Indian who developed himself by Yoga without a guru.

Wood, Ernest. *Practical Yoga*. Wilshire Book Co., 1972. An easily read exposition of Yogic philosophy by a recognized authority.

Swami Rama, et al. *Yoga Psychotherapy, the Evolution of Consciousness*. Himalayan Institute, Glenview, Illinois, 1976. A valuable book for the Yoga student or therapist who needs more knowledge in the other field to see the correlation. It presupposes some acquaintance with Yogic thought.

Swami Sivananda Radha. *The Divine Light Invocation: A Manual*. Ashram Press, Kootenay, Canada, 1966. Presents an ancient method for increasing awareness of the Light and its healing power. This may be obtained by writing to the Ashram.

ABOUT QUAKERS

Barbour, Hugh. *The Quakers in Puritan England*. Yale University Press, 1964. A good history of Quaker beginnings, including both their activities and ideas.

DuBois, Rachel Davis. *Deepening Quaker Faith and Practice Through the Use of the Three-Session Quaker Dialogue,* Ed. Mary Nankivel and Dorothy Ackerman, Ill. Eileen Brinton Waring. Friends United Press, Richmond, Indiana, 1976. Rachel applies her group dialogue technique to Meeting life in an outline with directions for Meeting use.

Hodgkin, L. Violet. *Quaker Saints*. T.N. Foulis, London, 1917. The story, "Fierce Feathers," is found in this book of Quaker tales, which has been reprinted in part many times.

London Yearly Meeting. *Christian Faith and Practice in the Experience of the Society of Friends*. Friends United Press, Richmond, Indiana, 1960. A modern re-working of *Faith and Practice,* the traditional handbook of the Society of Friends. It also includes many quotations on meditation and the Meeting for Worship.

Mack, Dorothy. "Clearness Committee," *Friends Journal,* August 1/15, 1974. A description of the way Meeting members can minister to each other, within our tradition and ability, in times of crisis and decision.

Zielinski, Stanislaw. *Psychology and Silence,* Pendle Hill Pamphlet #201. Wallingford, Pa., 1975. A thoughtful discussion of the phenomenon of Meeting for Worship.

About American Indians

Castaneda, Carlos. *The Teachings of Don Juan: A Yaqui Way of Knowledge.* University of California Press, 1968. A discussion of the "Man of Knowledge" and his four natural enemies shows dramatically the built-in obstacles to spiritual development.

Steiger, Brad. *Medicine Power.* Doubleday, New York, 1974. The Winnebago Indians' initiation, entitled "Vision Quest," tells of a spiritual opening to an adolescent boy.

―――――. *Medicine Talk,* Doubleday, New York, 1975. Twylah Nitche's description of the Senecas' approach to silent meditation is especially interesting to Friends.

General

Ackerman, Dorothy. "Opening the Door to Spiritual Awareness," *Friends Journal,* September 15, 1970.

Brown, Barbara. *New Mind, New Body, Biofeedback.* Harper and Row, New York, 1975. A complete survey of biofeedback research, including laboratory study of subjects in meditation.

Del Vasto, Lanzo. *Principles and Precepts of the Return to the Obvious.* Schocken Books, New York, 1974. The philosophy of a Catholic follower of Gandhi who is putting the teaching of Gandhi and Jesus into practice in his community in France.

Way of a Pilgrim, trans. R.M. French. Seabury Press, New York, 1972. A description of the use of mantra in the Christian tradition, from an ancient Russian manuscript, origin unknown.

Heard, Gerald. *Pain, Sex, and Time.* Harper & Brothers. New York, 1939. Interesting on meditation, but currently out of print.

_____. *Training for the Life of the Spirit,* Harper & Brothers, New York, 1941. Still valid, though written a generation ago.

Teilhard de Chardin, Pierre. *The Phenomenon of Man.* Harper & Brothers, New York, 1959. A scientist priest states a philosophy for the new age.

Thurman, Howard. *Mysticism and the Experience of Love,* Pendle Hill Pamphlet #115. Wallingford, Pa., 1961. The incident in the text of my pamphlet was told me personally by Howard Thurman; I have not seen it in print. He has written many devotional books based on his many years as a Protestant minister. *Deep Is the Hunger* and *Inward Journey* (Harper & Brothers) are my favorites.